PUNK
MEDICINE

DOING ITS BEST TO PROFIT THE MEDICAL INDUSTRY

PUNK MEDICINE
Copyright © 2022 by Dr. Robert J Brown

Published in the United States of America
ISBN   Paperback: 978-1-959165-36-1
ISBN   eBook: 978-1-959165-37-8

All rights reserved. No part of this publication may be reproduced, stored in a retrieval system or transmitted in any way by any means, electronic, mechanical, photocopy, recording or otherwise without the prior permission of the author except as provided by USA copyright law.

The opinions expressed by the author are not necessarily those of ReadersMagnet, LLC.

ReadersMagnet, LLC
10620 Treena Street, Suite 230 | San Diego, California, 92131 USA
1.619. 354. 2643 | www.readersmagnet.com

Book design copyright © 2022 by ReadersMagnet, LLC. All rights reserved.

Cover design by Ericka Obando
Interior design by Daniel Lopez

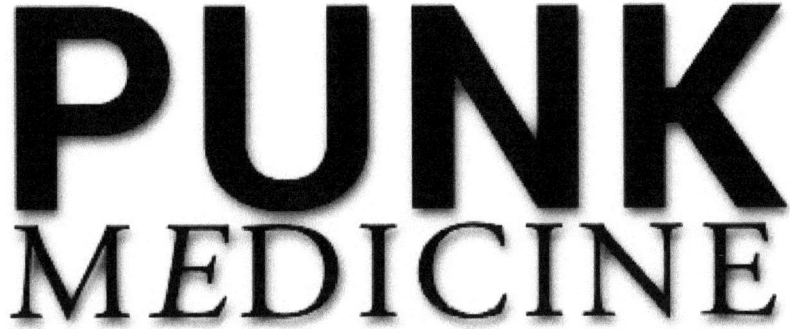

PUNK MEDICINE

DOING ITS BEST TO PROFIT THE MEDICAL INDUSTRY

Dr. Robert J Brown

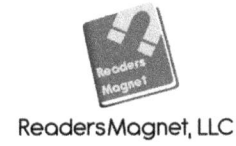

ReadersMagnet, LLC

PREFACE

I hope my first book inspired its readers to become a proactive part of their LIFE, HAPPINESS, AND HEALTHCARE. This book will reveal not only why you MUST be proactive, but what has caused this crisis of illegitimate science, inadequate medicine and government to get so out of control. Lobbying the FDA and the CDC should be illegal, but how can we get that past a congress that is heavily lobbied(bribed) and makes itself exempt from the laws they made for you and me to follow?

We are faced with seemingly endless corruption. In the name of profit, industries are allowed to commit acts that end up resulting in indirect mass murder and are supported by those whom we elected to prevent it. WHY? – GREED. This is nothing new and seems to have always been part of civilization. But now, the results are far more profound, causing pain, suffering, and death to millions throughout the world. The USA, who spends more on healthcare than any other country, is a failure when it comes to getting what it paid for.

Big Pharma doctors are treating symptoms — not patients — and are discouraged from learning any treatment that leaves big pharma and their profits out. Because these crooks have created many of the "standards of care" for medical treatment which are to be followed to avoid malpractice suits, doctors find themselves performing useless treatment or giving drugs just to comply with the standard. I, myself, have been prescribed drugs that were not necessary, with dangerous side effects, because it was the "standard of care."

Here are some examples of this greed. Pfizer took over a company that was developing the Milano Protein, which prevented arteries from developing plaque. Pfizer shut it down so they could make billions on Lipitor which can severely damage the liver. Moreover, it is not that effective. Pfizer took a discovery that had worked for centuries and replaced it with poorly researched crap.

A few years ago, the sugar industry was found to have bribed researchers at Harvard to supply "scientific" proof that saturated fats were the cause of heart disease. Not only is sugar a major factor in heart disease, but in most diseases. WHY is no one being made responsible for the mass murder resulting from this bribe? Even if no one suffered, the act of lying as an "expert," for profit, should be punishable.

In writing my first book, in addition to making the reader proactive in his healthcare, I wanted the reader to be aware that our government is NOT on our side. It is now unconstitutionally trying to politically force the people to follow medical practices that have not been properly researched or even proven to work. It is up to you and me to bring discipline to the medical industry. There are wonderful doctors and scientists making incredible breakthroughs in overcoming health problems that are being stopped by our FDA.

To quote Dr. Alan Sears in his medical letter "Confidential Cures," just look at the markup of these popular drugs:

- Celebrex (arthritis drug) – 21,712%
- Prilosec (heartburn) – 69,417 %
- Prozac (antidepressant) – 224,973 %

No one involved in our behemoth healthcare system… not Big Pharma, Big Medicine, or the FDA… wants you to have real cures. Their trillion-dollar cash cow would dry up.

You and I have to face criminal prosecution if we cause damage to another, yet government and industry seem to have no responsibility and answer to no one. The FDA and the CDC are overflowing with corruption. They are quite aware that they are preventing cures for cancer as well as other diseases. The CDC is forcing vaccinations on us that can do far more harm than good, but create a very healthy cash cow for their lobbyists. To avoid being prosecuted for helping these crooks, congress many times makes themselves exempt from their own laws. We had to accept Obamacare while the politicians had you and me buy them top private, medical insurance.

The mainstream media supports this corruption, for some reason, and almost never informed their followers of the real results, such as the death rates cause by vaccines, the actual death numbers due to Covid-19, or the true results of forcing unproven procedures on the public, or why certain cures we're not promoted including proper diet.

The normal flu seasons killed around 70,000 per year and this number drop to nothing during Covid.

Couldn't be the flu death where called Covid death since hospital death paid money for each Covid death? Africa has by far, tremendously lower Covid death rates in any other nations, without lockdowns, mask and social distancing. Why?

THE ROOT OF THE PROBLEM

What has caused man to become so self-destructive? Underlying everything in most men's thinking process is the EGO. Because of the ego, man can become greedy, selfish, defensive, offensive, possessive, destructive, and stressed, but, worse, detached from God. Our egos live in the left subjective brain and when you add the left-brain emphasis on subjective thinking, practiced by our educational system, one can become unable to "get outside the box" to see his own flaws. A very ugly, self-righteous, all-knowing, and judgmental individual, sometimes quite rich, with a desire to have control over others, can be a result.

What is the basic difference of left-brain dominance verses right? The left-brain-dominant person assumes he has a superior knowledge of many subjects, which creates the ultimate home in which the ego can thrive — subjective thinking. The right-brain-dominated person, not being dominated by ego, would feel his knowledge to be the equivalent of a few grains taken from a large mound of sand and that our total knowledge is almost worthless compared to what is to learn. The right-brained person is free to live creatively, is usually not as self-defensive and judgmental, and is much less led by memorized thoughts forced on us by our misguided educational system and the purposely biased media. Real problems are worked out in the right brain because it doesn't think it knows everything and seeks to find out how to solve the problems through objective thinking. Right brain wants a win-win game; left usually wants only to win at any cost.

This is an ancient problem with humanity. Even Buddha spent a great deal of time explaining the damage caused by our ego, and how to overcome it, to be able to enjoy so much more of life as a result of being truly open and free. The following is a writing, from Buddha's time, which expresses the opposite philosophy of what most of humanity embraces.

Be Thankful

Be thankful that you don't already have everything you desire. If you did, what would there be to look forward to?

Be thankful when you don't know something for it gives you the opportunity to learn.

Be thankful for the difficult times. During those times you grow.

Be thankful for each new challenge because it will build strength and character.

Be thankful for your mistakes. They will teach you valuable lessons.

Be thankful when you are tired and weary because it means you have made a difference.

It is easy to be thankful for good things.

A life of rich fulfillment comes to those who are also thankful for the setbacks.

> **Gratitude can turn a negative to a positive.**
>
> **Find a way to be thankful for your troubles and they become your blessings.**

The above was written over 2000 years ago and we think we progress over time? Today's spoiled brats want as much as they can get for as little as they can give — the peaks without the valleys. Actually, it is not just the young brats, but many rich old brats as well.

Much of our ego is formed when we are quite young and, as we age, we continue to rely on that child to guide our emotions. We go through our life being pushed around by this teenager's set of identity decisions. Dr. Wayne Dyer wrote of a heart surgeon he was treating for depression. He asked the surgeon what he would really enjoy doing as a profession.

The surgeon related that he was a nut for baseball statistics and would truly enjoy being an announcer. When Wayne asked him why he wasn't doing what he loved, he replied that he went through many years of training and expense to become what he is. Wayne asked him when he decided on that profession and he replied he decided when he was around 18. Dr. Dyer then asked him if he would go to an 18-year-old for advice on what to do for the rest of his life. The surgeon made the decision to change professions, becoming very successful in his favorite field, and is no longer depressed.

To best describe or identify ourselves, we use such words as I, me, and myself. Then we can further go into more description by adding adjectives, like I'm handsome, I'm smart, I'm good at what I do, or add greed and say I'm rich, I own a lot, or I control many. Then look in the dictionary and see how many pages of words begin with self, like selfish, self-image, self-abuse …. If we look from another perspective, these words represent very little as everything about us is in a constant state of change, not to mention they are words made to describe subjective opinions — judgments. It is like quantum conclusion. In quantum mechanics, one can only describe an electron for an instant of time. The very next instant, many changes can and do occur. Even though a dogmatic, left-brained person may fight change, the environment and conditions may, hopefully, force the old fart to think a new and different thought.

To prevent acknowledgment of such changes, we use our ego. We describe ourselves in such a manner that change is not allowed, at least for some time and, in some cases, a very long time. Our ego demands this, for change is very frightening to an ego. That little brat kid created it will defend it to the death, sometimes to the death of someone else or possibly disrupting his mind, causing a mental disorder. This character trait can seriously cause us to miss out on all other things that we could observe, if we allowed change. Instead, if ego driven, we are forced to exist in a static world. There can be joy, love, and beauty all around us and we see nothing that doesn't agree with "our world" as if there were a veil between us and reality. How depressing it becomes, and I use the word depressing literally — causing depression. Old age can result in spending one's last years in boredom reliving each day the same as the last. To stay vital and alive, one must seek newness and change.

"THE VEILS OF EGO" is a term introduced by Mathieu Recard in his book "Happiness." These veils can make the viewer see only what is expected and prevents seeing situations of beauty, love, and kindness and GOD. Example: *That kind of person can't be trusted and should not be in my world.* That person is Jesus.

Needless to say, our self-image can be designed by our ego which can create selfishness and greed. We compete to have more possessions, to have a newer car, to get better grades, to be in better shape, to have more friends, and to make more money. There is nothing wrong with these achievements, but they should only come as a result of helping others, making our world a better place, or win-win relationships — NOT AFTER YOU ACHIEVE YOUR GOAL, BUT IN THE PROCESS OF ACHIEVING IT. In the process of helping others, such as a doctor making his patients' health better, achieving of that goal helps to lessen the strangle hold the ego has. It is wonderful to create wealth by making others win, plus it can bolster real self-esteem and integrity, which the greedy takers lost long ago. Our creator has an endless supply of LOVE for us to share with our fellowmen. The ideal world is a world where all deserving beings win.

My deep philosophical belief is that THE PURPOSE OF LIFE IS LOVE. You will find that when you get your life into an emotional mess, you most likely have been off PURPOSE. Everything a *truly* successful person does is meant to benefit others. Quantum mechanics explains that we think and communicate GOD'S way so that, to a certain extent, we may become GOD in a very quantum way, quantum being the smallest particle that exists.

Recently, quantum has directed me to change negative thoughts into positive, a very logical move since negative thoughts tend to be subjective and judgmental. I have found it is like getting the traditional monkey off my back to avoid negative thinking, for who am I to determine what is good or bad? After all, Ecc. 3:1 states that *there is a time for everything…*

The work of Dr. Bethany Kok, at the University of North Carolina, called "Project Bless," clearly demonstrates that a giving and loving attitude can improve one's health by stimulating the vagus nerve which controls the parasympathetic nervous system, the opposite of the fight-or-flight system, the sympathetic nervous system. Arousing the parasympathetic nervous system brings improved function to all of our organs along with fulfillment and peace to our minds. Thus, one might say the selfishness of an egocentric person can bring that person stress and poor health. This agrees with quantum physics, which many researchers feel comes directly from GOD. If an idea has anything to do with one's opinion, is subjective, GOD is not involved. If a statement does not come from love, GOD is not involved.

It was discovered recently that our heart has brain cells which think more like GOD and are activated to communicate with our brain by a state of parasympathetic dominance. Only then will it communicate with our conscience brain. This has given us answers to many mysteries. How have the philosophers, poets, and song writers known about this for centuries?

Matthieu Recard, in his book, "Happiness," clearly tells us how to get out from under the control of this monster thing called ego, which is actually a young spoiled brat, or possibly, an insecure underachiever or criminal, due to a poor self-image. I have referred many of my pain clinic patients to read this book to help them manage stress, with fabulous results.

It has been said that the "love of money is the root of all evil." I wish that were all. Let's add "craving for power is a root of all evil." Why do billionaires want more, many times causing others to suffer and die? Many try to push their political agenda on you and me to maintain their power or promote their ideas. A part of the answer is found in Dr. Dyer's book "Secrets of Manifesting" in which he points out six factors of ego, the sixth being denial of GOD.

In this chapter, I hope not only to enrich your life, but to get you to understand what you need, not only to deny information from "qualified sources", but be very suspicious of why you are advised to do whatever is recommended by the "standard of care" that guides doctors and the establishment. My reason for bringing the benefits of quantum and Godly philosophies into punk medicine is that, like Dr. Samanta-Laughton explains, science has been punk science because GOD was left out. Medicine has become punk medicine for the same reasons. There are multiple cures that have been purposely forgotten, avoided, or made illegal for ungodly reasons, mostly greed and arrogance.

To further the complexity of trying to correct our medical dilemma, our society likes to put doctors on a pedestal, or "ivory tower" depending on the size of the doctor's ego, making the doctor feel like he is the ultimate authority on most subjects of healthcare. My last NDE was these "authorities" concluding I needed the covid vaccine. They assumed the anti-antibody treatment for Guillian Barre required the stimulation of more covid-19 antibodies. Due to the subjective methods of the education in medical schools, teaching the brain to think only of drugs to treat illnesses, many are limited to spitting out memorized treatment methods without applying reason, but they are within the "standard of care" and protected from litigation. Result: I got to spend three days of being very close to death and my family got to suffer along.

CHAPTER 1

Most of the medical establishments assume the current aging process is normal — getting old by 60, cutting back on physical activity and requiring assistance in the 70's, losing brain function in the 80's, along with more physical disabilities and dying in the 90's or earlier. When I see what older people eat, I can see they are forced into the bogus aging expectations their doctors suggest. Add their little plastic, flip-top box full of pills, with the time and day they must take them, with their side effects, and you have a disaster in progress.

Since I changed to a Paleo diet, adding several supplements to overcome our poor farming and modern food preservation, I am getting younger and enjoying the best health of my life. Even though I look and act 10 to 30 years younger than some of my patients, they are already committed to the status quo. I do inspire many to change and the results are wonderful. TO TRULY ENJOY BECOMING OLDER AND NOT AGING, THE CURENT "STANDARD OF CARE" MUST BE CHALLENGED.

Dr. David Sinclair of Harvard lectures on this subject, stating that we should, at 150 years, be acting more like those in their 60's. When you stop a physical activity, like swimming, the nerve connections to create those muscle performances deteriorate and the muscles atrophy. The same occurs with the brain. Even some fasting helps you to age more slowly. Medications can accelerate aging by covering up symptoms caused by bad habits and destroying mitochondria. Future chapters will explain the vital function of mitochondria in all functions of our bodies and in our health and vitality.

A SYMPTOM IS YOUR BODY CRYING OUT FOR HELP. THE DRUG, no, the doctor, IS SAYING SHUT UP and take this!!

Masking the symptom can allow what is causing it to continue its destruction.

LIFESTYLE, ATTITUDE, AND DIETARY CHANGES, PLUS PROPER SUPPLEMENTS, PLUS PROPER APPLICATION OF ALTERNATIVE AND ANCIENT MEDICINE, CAN TREAT PATIENTS WITH ONLY BENEFICIAL SIDE EFFECTS.

Drugs, surgery, and radiation should be a last resort — well after trying alternative approaches — but there is simply too much profit made selling drugs plus the patient will always need more or different drugs for the side effects. One of my patients was scheduled for a hip replacement. Her diet was average — in other words, very deficient. With my guidance, she changed her diet to an anti-inflammatory diet and supplemented with highly anti-inflammatory and antioxidant supplements, NOT DRUGS. She noticed almost immediate improvement, and cancelled the surgery. Three years have passed with no further symptoms.

In my practice, this has become a profound method of choice with consistent results. The only difficult problem is you are not allowed to satisfy your craving for sugar which never ends unless you stop it. This holistic approach requires a much more educated and creative doctor, requiring much more knowledge and understanding of the patient as well as basic sciences and psychology. In my lectures, I mention that one of the most important medical books that has helped my holistic approach to medicine is "How to Win Friends and Influence People" by Dale Carnegie. I take a lot of time on my initial exam because I want the patient to think of me as a friend and someone they can really trust. My conversations center on the patient's life and favorite subjects, along with the problem that brought them in. Unless we become friends, how can I ever get them to stop their favorite foods and begin a healthy lifestyle? In many cases, within a few days of initiating my treatment, my patients are excited and become an active part of their treatment.

By an incredible coincidence, today I got a call from a patient that had been suffering myoclonus (uncontrollable twitching of her soft palate) for ten years. She had tried every field of medicine, from botox injections to neurology and other fields. Being told there was nothing that medicine could do, she came to me because she learned I was in alternative medicine. My normal treatment method was useless so I dismissed telling her that I would make this a research project. My premedical training was a major in physiology with minors in chemistry and biochemistry. Physiology taught me that involuntary muscle activity can originate from the cerebral cortex and my knowledge of chemistry indicated that magnesium had the side effect of calming this activity. Now getting Mg through the blood brain barrier is most easily done using Mg L-Threonate. To get the highest concentration quickly, put the powder under the tongue. Hit the nerve at each end.

The call I got today was my patient calling to tell me that the ten years of misery is over.

CHAPTER 2

THE MEDICAL ESTABLISHMENT
HOW THEY STOP PROGRESS FOR POWER AND PROFIT

*"If we knew what it was we were doing,
it would not be called research, would it?"*
—Albert Einstein

There have been, throughout history, incredible discoveries that would have advanced science and healthcare immensely. Up pops the ego and greed of the establishment and these discoveries are trashed and even degraded. In several cases, the doctor's inventions were put in the Museum of Medical Quackery, only to find much later they were creations of genius. The medical industry has stopped at nothing to discredit homeopathy. They took their efforts to the extreme extent of murdering alternative doctors.

In another industry, look what happened to Nikola Tesla. Among many things Tesla discovered was how to get free electricity without the associated pollution we now suffer. Can you imagine the trillions of dollars industry would have not made if they had not succeeded in destroying him and his work? Can you also imagine what a wonderful world we would have if we could throw off one of the ego's favorite personality traits, GREED, plus, eliminate two other ego character traits, the desire for recognition and the craving for power? We would be approaching nirvana.

Many great discoveries in medicine have been condemned and discarded by the "leaders in the field" as quackery. A classic case, from over 100 years ago, was the discoveries and inventions of Dr. Albert Abrams. "Science" was finally accepting the discovery of the atom as being mostly electricity, but was hanging on to not allowing this to be applied to living organs that you and I possess.

Dr. Adams was quite wealthy due to family inheritance. When he completed medical school here, with honors, he learned the German language and went on to double his qualifications at the University of Heidelberg, earning the respect of the great doctors of Europe. Returning to San Francisco, he became Director of Medical Studies at Stanford University. This was at the time that the atomic theory was coming to life. Dr. Abrams was among the first to apply this theory to medicine.

Each atom or element has characteristic numbers of protons and electrons which give them their properties. Each gives off a characteristic wave signature which can be detected. Abrams believed that different tissues could also be identified by their characteristic electromagnetically-based signatures and that diseased and degenerated tissues could also emit a unique electrical phenomenon.

In around 1916, Abrams wrote the following declaration:

> *"As physicians we dare not stand aloof from the recent amazing advances made in Physical Science, and segregate the human entity from other entities of the physical universe whether the object of our differentiation is a healthy man, or merely a mass of diseased tissue. We are, in either case, dealing only with a congregation of vibrant atoms, which in their innumerable molecular combinations, are the basic constituents of everything that exists."*

One can just imagine how this was received. Needless to say, his declaration did not receive the slightest bit of interest from the medical establishment and I'm sure he was not well-liked by the religious community.

To our good fortune, Dr. Abrams did not have to raise money and funded a very elaborate laboratory, attracting scientists from the physical sciences. One of which was Samuel Hoffman, an acknowledged inventor in the infant field of radio.

Little, if anything, was known on how to detect very small emissions produced by atomic and molecular vibrations. Abrams and Hoffman were the first to use the rheostat in medicine to change frequencies of magnetic radiation and its detection. The emissions were so minute that they could only be detected when the patient faced west so that the earth's magnetic field would not interfere. The science originated by

Abrams is today referred to as radionics. The instruments he invented were called the reflexophone and oscilloclast.

Dr. Abrams was able to detect many diseases, including cancer, with his method, well before the established methods could come close and, in many cases, haven't yet. There is a lot more to his story that, with effort, one can find on the internet, including the emotional beating Dr. Abrams took from the establishment which put his inventions to be displayed in a museum of medical quackery. This genius ended his career in disgrace, referred to by the medical profession as "a charlatan, a quack, and shameless exploiter of the sick and suffering for the sake of financial gain." That last statement more describes much of our pharmaceutical industry and Abram's critics.

There is much more to the Abrams research. He found that a drug that treated a disease like malaria, quinine, has electromagnetic emission that can destroy the disease without the chemical coming in contact with the diseased tissue. This helps explain homeopathic medicine, which the establishment, even now, laughs at. Properly applied, this could open the door to using new drugs that, if injected, have too many side effects such as death, but their electromagnetic energy could be used instead. A century later, true scientists are finally rediscovering new methods of diagnosis and treatment that should have been developed decades ago had the establishment not prevent it.

I recently traveled to Budapest where I went to learn about a Russian device that can detect problems in our organs well in advance of a disease. I was quite pleased to have the technicians inquire into my diet and lifestyle because my organs tested out to be far younger than my age, but if they found a distressed organ, it could be corrected preventively or at least we could work on the cause and strengthen that organ accordingly.

Shortly after the death of Dr Abrams, another genius, Royal Raymond Rife appeared, not a physician, but a genius in the field of technology, famous for developing a 2700-horsepower marine engine in 1915. Another Rife invention was a 50,000 power microscope which used quartz prisms in a glycerin bath. The best modern science can do doesn't come close. We now get even higher magnification with the electron microscope, but the electron microscope can only study dead tissue samples. Can you imagine the stupidity of "modern medicine" to not prefer Rife's microscope?

He could watch how TB bacteria died, splitting into even smaller living particles he called TB viruses. We call this pleomorphism, which today is bitterly disputed. Those who challenge his findings have never looked through his microscope. Rife was the first to ever see and study living viruses. Rife possessed one of Abram's oscilloclasts and redesigned it to generate a wider spectrum of individual frequencies which revealed even more astounding information. He found that if you direct a certain resonate frequency at an organism, it will vibrate until it bursts — like a singer can break a glass. This is true for pathogens and cancer cells. He determined 600 different frequencies for various organisms which he termed the MOR or mortal oscillatory rate.

In 1935, Rife gathered 16 terminally ill cancer and TB patients, exposed each of them to the proper frequency for their pathogen or diseased cells. After 70 days, there were 14 cured and the other two recovered completely shortly after. NO DRUGS USED! No one could achieve that now and yet most continue to refute it.

Although Rife received numerous international awards for his achievements and was honored with a medical degree from Heidelberg University in Germany, he is considered a quack by the USA establishment, his machines made illegal, and lab destroyed. This is rumored by the FDA. Much of the push to destroy Rife and his inventions came from the leaders of the medical profession who saw the possibility of taking over his company and making a fortune. He would not give in. Thus, we are denied the ability to cure terrible diseases without medications, which many times fail and have horrible side effects.

You don't need to go back as far as Rife's time to find even worse crimes done by the medical establishment, which includes the pharmaceutical industry, the medical industry, the hospital industry, and the political complex including FDA, CDC, EPA and the USDA. It is speculated that over 100 alternative doctors have been murdered in the recent years. One who survived was Dr. Sam Chachoua. Dr. Chachoua is a genius of our time who has discovered a powerful treatment for both cancer and AIDS. His work is so important that it was plagiarized by much respected institutions, who want to take credit for it, and yet, at the same time, they condemn it. His methods are so revolutionary and successful that he is a threat to the status quo and they are quite afraid of losing their hold on the profits. The establishment is worried that you and I might profit by not suffering at their hands. Dr. Oz and Martin Sheen have also condemned Dr.

Chachoua. Listen to Chachoua's side of the story on the net and see how totally anti-intellectual our society has become, and it appears to be getting worse. When Chachoua first presented his discoveries, a very renowned institution, Cedars-Sanai, was so impressed that they announced the cure was here. Shortly after, Cedars destroyed all of Chachoua's serums and denounced his work. I'd like to follow the money on this one. Chachoua won a 10 million dollar legal action, but that's pocket change to big pharms. To quote Edward Deming, "A bad system will beat a good person every time."

> *Each progressive spirit is opposed by a thousand mediocre minds appointed to guard the past.*
>
> —Maurice Maeterlinck

FAKE SCIENCE is another tool the establishment uses in order to retard progress and promote profits. Recently, scientists at the University of California San Francisco Medical center exposed two fake scientists at Harvard, who were bribed by the sugar industry to make us believe fats were the main cause of heart disease when the real culprit is sugar. I'm surprised Pfizer wasn't in on it to help support the questionable benefits of Lipitor.

As a graduate student, I was the recipient of several research fellowships. In many cases I was assigned the grunt work of reviewing the literature for the professors leading the projects. I quickly found that not all research is valid. One clue is what my Einstein quote above is about. The researchers were not doing research; they were trying to justify and prove predetermined beliefs. Time after time a misconception was justified and falsely reestablished by biased "scientists." Example: You can breed a laboratory animal to be so sensitive and cancer-prone that almost anything it is given will cause cancer. A researcher can purposely ignore or destroy findings that disagree with what he was hired to prove. A pharmaceutical company can employ scientists to monitor the work of other scientists who may be into discovering something that would cut into their monopoly. I personally know a doctor who was working on peptide research to cure cancer with three others. They were given ten million dollars to discontinue their work and made to sign an agreement to stay out of that field. They were all in their twenties and that's quite a chunk of money.

To exacerbate the problem, the term "evidence based" has become a requirement for lecturers to adhere to in presenting their subject at medical schools and seminars. "Evidence based" information is hypocrisy if you consider the junk science it is based on.

There are many diseases caused by poor diet and lifestyle. Over fifty years ago, Dr. Colon Dong wrote a book entitled "New Hope for the Arthritic". In this book there are many testimonials of patients who were bedridden with arthritis and were able to assume a normal life through diet alone. Arthritis doctors, rheumatologists, rarely emphasize diet, going immediately to drugs to lessen the pain and decrease inflammation. After all, big money controls what these specialists are taught in a drug-treatment-dominated medical school. At the expense of repeating myself, this approach is like giving pain meds and anti-inflammatory drugs for a thorn in your foot. The pain may be lessened, but the damage continues. Once again the symptom was treated, not the patient. For several years now, real doctors have known that stimulating the vagus nerve can greatly lessen the effects of rheumatoid arthritis and many other autoimmune diseases, but the "standard of care" has yet to recognize this protocol. There are no side effects to microcurrent therapy, one method of vagus stimulation, but the medical establishment dictates the "standard of care," preferring drugs with serious potential side effects, including death, as the treatment.

Another abuse delivered by medical practitioners is total neglect of our immune system in the prevention of diseases, using antibiotics to treat many of them. The side effects of antibiotics can be extremely painful, debilitating, and deadly. The abuse of these drugs can lead to making the patient susceptible to other infectious diseases in addition to destroying the very important flora of bacteria in our intestines, potentially leading to colon cancer and recently discovered cognitive problems. In addition, the abuse of these drugs can result in resistant bacteria as well as not allowing our immune system to develop the identity of the germ into its "memory banks" for future defense.

Let us never forget that "SCIENCE" IS NOT FACT. I highly recommend the book "PUNK SCIENCE" by Dr. Manjir Samantha-Laughton. She explains what causes science to change opinions on many "facts," sometimes radically, at regular intervals. There is no such thing as "Pure Science". Man does not have a brain that has evolved enough to understand perfectly his own creation or, much less, get his ego out of the way enough to seek the truth. We have cures or much better treatments for many diseases but the multi trillion-dollar cash cows will do anything to stay in control.

CHAPTER 3

The Magnificent Immune System

Consider your body like a house. Take the locks off the doors, eliminate the lights, telephone, defense weapons, and police. How do you prevent the bad guys from taking over? It would literally be HELL! Whenever a group of criminals happened by, you lose. There is never peace. You can hire strong guys to beat up the bad guys, but it's expensive, keeping you from using your money for fun and improvement or even going to the store for food. If the utilities, such as water and sewer are not dependable, the internal problem gets out of control. I could go at length about the misery you would experience. To be honest with you, that is what many of us do with our bodies. Unless you are one of the followers of my last book or have researched yourself on lifestyle, diet, and attitude, you have very little defense against sickness. Run to the strong guys, doctors, use drugs to beat up the bad guys and live with poor utilities. THIS DOES NOT HAVE

TO HAPPEN. YOU CAN MOVE TO "ALMOST HEAVEN", a great place to live.

The germ theory of disease misses the real phenomena creating this dysfunction. Our bodies are not just made up of cells. There are complex systems, including bacteria that service those cells, just like you service a home. There must be supply routes bringing supplies and sewers, taking the waste out as well as energy to make organs function. When we put processed foods and chemicals into the supply line of our body, along with adding pollution through breathing, drinking, electromagnetic exposure, and drugs, we can seriously clog up supply lines and the sewer. Then add stress, which multiplies these problems and one can seriously stop certain cellular activity that creates whatever cleansing is possible. The result is you have a neighborhood where your healthy cells can no longer exist.

One classic example of clogging the sewer through diet and lifestyle is found in the brain. Glial cells are found among our neurons. There are several types of glial cells which act to pad and protect neurons like styrofoam pads protect a box of fine crystal. Unless your sleep is very good, going through REM into delta, where the body is still enough, these cells can't do an important function. That function is to shrink to 1/10 their size, allowing the fluids in the brain to be exchanged, removing toxins, such as MSG plus cellular waste. If you don't go into deep sleep, you get to enjoy your foggy, forgetful brain, and the next morning coffee won't cure the damage. If you add the chemicals in processed foods that can pass the blood-brain barrier, you clog what drainage there is (the sewer), so even if the glial cells work, the waste can't be disposed of.

I would like to propose what happens when cleansing cannot occur. Others before me have proposed similar beliefs, but it is yet to become acknowledged. When the garbage is allowed to build within cellular systems the polluted fluids can cause an altering of the electromagnetic signatures of the cells, resulting in degeneration or mutation and loss of communication with other cells. Chronic inflammation usually occurs as well, further exacerbating the dilemma. We now have produced an engraved, gold-lettered invitation to pathogens to come into our body and have encouraged our cells to no longer communicate with each other. Now they can join other cancer cells and go about their merry way with no supervision. This polluted environment inhibits the ability of our immune cells to fight for us, allowing the disease to get a good foothold before surrounding the disease with hopefully healthy cells that can take up the battle. SUGAR alone can be like throwing gasoline into a fire when it comes to destroying our immune system plus slowing down vital cells.

INFLAMMATION is the number one cause of most diseases. Medical schools teach that it is a result of the infection. THE MAJOR CAUSE OF INFLAMMATION IS DIETARY. "ITIS" is a suffix which means inflammation—ie: gingivitis – inflammation of the gums, colitis - inflammation of the colon, and arthritis-inflammation of a joint. "Modern medicine" has a treatment, a drug, or surgery, for most "itises" with some really bad side effects. As you will find further in this book, there are much more successful methods, some around for centuries and some now being developed, to allow one to use one's own immune system to stop inflammation. In fact, recent research has unchallengeable findings that if the brain is cared for properly, it can be like a third immune system directing the production of many products that can fight for us, even curing cancer.

Below is a list of anti-inflammatory practices that can decrease your susceptibility to disease, possibly ending common diseases entirely.

- Become proactive in learning everything you can about how you can achieve all that you want from this wonderful opportunity called life. Include the study of newly developing quantum medicine.
- Learn about the anti-inflammatory index and the foods you need to counteract inflammation. Install an inflammatory and an anti-inflammatory index application for your smart phone.
- Learn the inflammatory index so as to avoid eating certain foods, like sugar, rice, starch, and whole grains.
- Stay as close to nature as possible, including walking barefoot on earth a little, to ground yourself. Processed foods, such as breakfast cereal, can contain Roundup, BHA, and BHT. "Natural seasonings" on a label can mean MSG. Our enemy, the FDA, allows MSG to be called natural flavorings and BHA and BHT to be dusted in a box of cereal which doesn't require it on the label.
- Study using supplements to make up for the fact that we can't get important nutrients that we evolved with. Until quite recently we had no refrigeration and much of our food was spoiled creating beneficial nutrients we can no longer obtain.
- Don't follow the USDA or any other government source of dietary information. Do you consult a politician for health advice? The food pyramid, if followed, can cause many health problems, some very serious. Hopefully, someday, we will end lobbying(legalized bribery), eliminating a big factor in the creation of crooked politicians.
- Beware of fad diets. It is best to educate yourself and create your own personal diet. I will get into that as well as proper

- supplements in a future chapter. A book by Dr. Keith Scott-Mumby, "Diet Wise," is quite informative and helpful to use in creating your personal diet.
- Learn about how you maintain an ideal intestinal flora. The typical American diet promotes a yeast, Candida, to dominate one's flora, creating sugar cravings. The resulting incomplete digestion (malnutrition) causes weight gain and poor health. You have all heard of probiotics, but do you also take prebiotics? Not adding the latter is like sending solders into battle without food.
- There is a test for inflammation, the CRP (C- reactive protein) that should be part of every physical exam. If it is not, find another doctor. This test can be of extreme importance.
- Avoid grain-fed meat and whole grains which are a direct cause of generalized inflammation. Whole grains contain lectin and gluten — poisons. Humans and their animals are the world's only grain eaters and not part of our evolution. The book "Grain Brain" by David Perlmutter, MD clearly points out the dangers of whole grains in our diet.
- Take supplements that enhance the immune system and help cleansing such as D3K2, NAC (N-acetyl-L-cysteine), AFA (from Blue-green algae), and Turmeric Curcumin to mention just a few.
- GET GOOD SLEEP!! We evolved with only candle and fire light(red tones). Blue light was to wake us up in the morning. Cell phones, computers, and TV are sleep preventers. Eating too late can interfere.
- CONTROL STRESS — it is easier than you think, using quantum mechanics.
- GOD gave us an incredible body capable of being able to fight off most diseases, IF WE EAT HIS FOOD.

There are many more practices, but these are a good start.

There is category of drugs called **immunosuppressant drugs**. Designed to suppress our only defense against disease, they are used, in many cases, as a short cut for the doctor to treat a symptom rather than the patient. Sure, the patient gets some relief, but the underlying cause is not diagnosed, so, as far as the disease is concerned, it can continue to worsen while the patient doesn't suffer quite so much, but will likely suffer a lot more later. Yes, these drugs are useful in preventing rejection of organ transplants and are, in these cases, necessary. Using them because the doctor is not up on new research and wants a quick fix or is just too lazy or busy to take the time to find the cause for your discomfort is no excuse.

Here are a few diseases, actually symptoms, treated with immunosuppressant drugs: Psoriasis = a skin rash that can be a food allergy or gluten intolerance symptom. Lupus – an autoimmune disease that has found to be treatable with microcurrent therapy (not approved in USA, but is in Europe). Rheumatoid arthritis- very successfully treated with microcurrent therapy in Europe. Crohn's disease- again, a symptom of a disease, the underlying cause should be sought. I have arrested every case of Crohn's I have seen in my office by working with an alternative specialist to find the food sensitivity or flora imbalance that was the underlying cause. I'm sure there may be other causes, but doctors, get off your asses and find them because Prednisone, one of the drugs of choice and "standard of care," is a dangerous drug with horrible side effects.

So many auto immune diseases (there are a very large number) are now being associated with the lack of activity of the vagus nerve. This can easily be tested. With **no side effects** microcurrent therapy can be applied to the nerve, sometime with immediate results, but not approved in the USA. WHY? All drugs in this category have bad side effects, sometimes fatal, but they are approved. WHY? Big Pharma's cash cow.

Having read numerous articles on managing inflammation with immunosuppressant drugs, I have yet to find in mainstream medical articles any mention of diet and supplements. For years, in my practice and those practices of holistic colleagues, we have routinely controlled inflammation with diet and supplementation. There are some foods like tart cherry juice and supplements like omega3 fatty acids that are profound anti-inflammatories. Just getting sugar, high glycemic foods, and additives out of the diet, along with grain-fed meats, can reduce inflammatory pain. Did you know that many of the farmed fish are fed grains? Atlantic salmon thus becomes a source of grain.

I have applied microcurrent therapy to areas of pain and inflammation to see the patient's mouth drop open in amazement when it disappears, sometimes after years of suffering. It has no side effects but has not been considered a "standard of care" or even approved.

We have a profound immune system which should be preserved and protected. No one knows how many cancers are destroyed each day by this wonderful system and yet our present chemotherapy and radiation treatments for cancer destroy the immune system. In Texas, Dr. Burzynski cures brain cancer using our own immune system. He has found that attaching peptides, called antineoplastons, to cancer cells, our immune cells recognize them, as foreign bodies and proceed to destroy them. No hospitals are necessary for his patients are taught to treat themselves. With hundreds of cured patients, who were given a death sentence by the "standard of care," the medical establishment has shown its gratitude by threatening him with multimillion dollar fines and multiple trials. One just finished recently in which he prevailed. Not much has changed since Abrams and Rife in the 1920's and 30's — still the same old egotistical establishment trying to preserve the past. A movie about Burzynski is available on the net.

What we understand now is that our immune system is made up of two very different systems: the Innate and the Adaptive immune systems. The first is automatic and the first line of defense, designed to "set off the alarm" and "fire the first shots." These responses are chemicals capable of not only killing the pathogen, but the host as well. In fact, the result is the autoimmune disease called Guillian-Barre syndrome. Toxic shock, a major cause of death in cancer victims, can be due to these chemicals.

The adaptive system is like our computer banks which contain the information about the pathogen and guide our "killer cells," — the lymphocytes, erythrocytes, megakaryocytes, and more, to destroy the now identified cell. Sometimes a pathogen has invaded and is within the cells. Destroying these requires an active and successful adaptive immune system which requires ideal conditions of nutrition and lifestyle. As mentioned above, quantum science has just discovered that the healthy and properly trained brain can be a third immune system.

As I mentioned before, science can create laboratory animals whose immune system is so degraded that usually normal foods and chemicals can stimulate cancer. A human can achieve that condition through self-abuse to the point that some vegetables may not be consumed. The work of Dr. Stephen Gundry, former cardiologist at Loma Linda Medical School, in his book "Plant Paradox," clearly demonstrates this condition. How to work on diet, supplementation, and lifestyle to avoid this horrible condition will be the subject of a future chapter.

CHAPTER 4

LEARNING FROM ANTIQUITY

"ONE THING I KNOW, AND THAT IS THAT I KNOW NOTHING"

—Socrates 399 BC

In the case of most professors and scientists you will rarely find this form of intelligence and humility – instead you will find the left brain dominant and egocentric attitude. The medical establishment has decided that science has progressed such that that the ideas of the past are not worth consideration. Plus industry can't profit on a cure they can't patent. We could all learn from Socrates. Einstein also had this philosophy. As I learned from Warner Earhart many years ago, "the truly brilliant minds realize they don't even know what they don't know". For me, realizing how infinite it is that I have yet to learn makes life even more magnificent. I have pity for those who have locked themselves in the all-knowing box and it seems that the more degrees they have after their name, the stronger their box is locked, although one PhD seems to be enough to grow the ego. To quote Isaac Asimov, "The true delight is finding out rather than knowing."THE DESTRUCTIVE ARROGANCE OF MAN is the key to why we are in so much trouble. Arrogantly, our medical leaders and scientists throw out the knowledge of previous generations thinking that modern is better. As I mentioned earlier, one of the characteristics of ego dominance is loss of belief in GOD. In fact, throwing out the knowledge of our predecessors, especially when many of their methods were successful, could be considered similar to thinking they are smarter than GOD. No one can ever determine whether or not previous methods were not directly given to us by our creator. Our creator made us far more able to survive than "modern medicine" has been able to if we eat HIS food. In fact, many primitive societies survive to be quite old, without doctors, by not eating our society's food or drugs.

Today I had a chance to relax and meditate in the sun. Watching the insects, I experienced an epiphany. Man cannot come close to the flying abilities of a fly or a butterfly or the energy of an ant. How can that tiny head contain enough brain to accomplish these abilities? Maybe it is not a brain, but DNA, which does have the configuration of a cell phone antenna, and could be receiving information from elsewhere. It is believed by many that our thoughts are not created inside our head, but somewhere in space. It has been proven that some vegetation can feel our emotions. This would explain out of body experiences and premonitions.

In my conversations with many very brilliant scientists, there is just too much evidence that humans were visited by aliens far more advanced than we, somewhere between four and ten thousand years ago. According to many, those visits have not yet been discontinued. The practice of acupuncture suddenly appeared thousands of years ago which required an advanced knowledge of the human body. "Modern science" continues to challenge acupuncture or just ignore it.

In 1971 the Father of American Cardiology and Nobel Prize winner, Paul Dudley White, returned from China where he had personally witnessed complex surgeries being performed using acupuncture only, without anesthesia or drugs. Sometimes a tranquilizer was given. The patient was able to have conversation while being worked on and able to walk to his hospital bed. Dr. White felt strongly that American medicine should replace life threatening anesthesia with acupuncture. The establishment refused to do so and prefers to kill innocent patients rather than sacrifice their cash cow. A friend of mine lost his wife to anesthesia merely having plastic surgery. "Modern medicine" has been around for around 100 years as opposed to over 4000 years for acupuncture. Greed and arrogance win again.

Another eastern medicine that has been around for thousands of years is Ayurveda — Ayurvedic Medicine. It was developed over three thousand years ago in India. It is based on the belief that our health depends on a delicate balance of, not just diet and lifestyle, but mind, spirit, and body. Early quantum? Unlike western, "modern," medicine, Ayurveda emphasizes the importance of the mind in bringing the body into balance. Freedom from disease requires expansion of one's awareness to refresh and restore balance. To accomplish this, the practice of quiet meditation, which brings us to a state of restful awareness, is necessary. Correction of a dysfunction in the performance of an organ requires our brain to be aware of the problem that the organ is experiencing. In our complex world, made worse by the fact that we are stressing ourselves over trivial pursuits, our brains are so wound up in our nonsense that to allow the brain to acknowledge a health problem requires that we enter an "alpha" state (meditative state) to remove nonsensical thought patterns, giving the brain freedom to attend to the needs of our body. Recent developments in the field of microcurrent therapy have used this ancient approach to create miracles in the elimination of pain and dysfunction. This new field also has learned from ancient acupuncture how to use, even more efficiently, microcurrent instead of needles.

The practice of Quantum Medicine uses brain control to cure most diseases and conditions. One can learn extensively on YouTube about this miracle by just searching YouTube for "Quantum Mechanics" and "Quantum Medicine". I highly recommend "Becoming Supernatural" by Dr. Joe Dispenza.

Another very important factor overlooked for decades by "modern medicine" is the ancient knowledge that our organs communicate with each other not just through the nervous system, but through the fascia. Fascia is a connective tissue which connects and supports every organ in our body and is the media through which acupuncture transmits its communication and stimulation. It is even found in bone. Learning from antiquity has resulted in the ability of microcurrent therapy to not only accelerate the healing process of our tissues, but, as one example, to allow horses to not be shot upon breaking a leg.

THE ASSEMBLAGE POINT AND CRYSTAL LIGHT THERAPY

Here's to all you extraterrestrial believers. Again, thousands of years ago, only this time all over the world appeared the Assemblage Point and Crystal Light Therapy. From Mayans and Incas and Native American Indians to East Indian Ayurvedics, healers used the power of healing crystals in their techniques. Below is a diagram of the energy fields associated with the ideally located assemblage point. In the patient, the exact location of the assemblage point can have a direct effect on a person's energy and is directly linked to all of the organs, affecting them directly. Again we return to quantum physics; the human body is an oscillating energy field with an epicenter which is referred to as the assemblage point. We can only speculate what communication with outside sources may occur. One factor that has been passed down from antiquity is there are many problems associated with the displacement of the assemblage point.

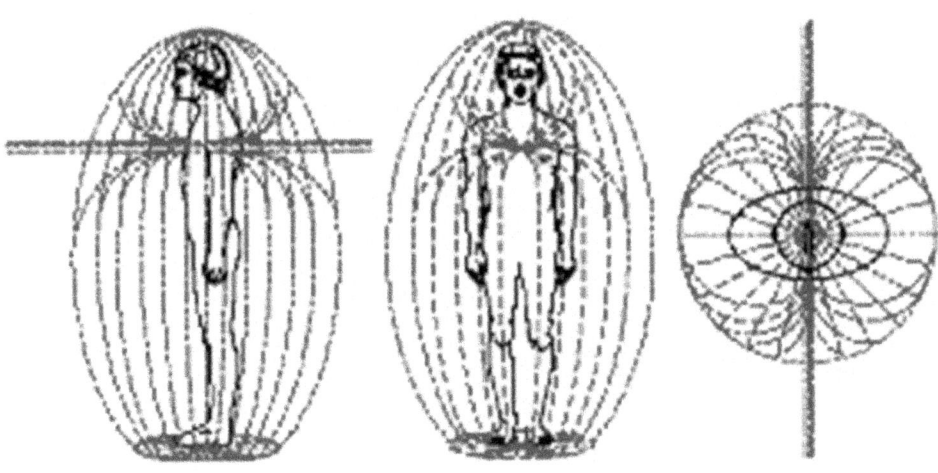

There are many reasons for the assemblage point (AP) to be out of position. Shock, trauma, stress, childhood abuse, and poor lifestyles are among them. Excessive left brain activity can move the AP to the right. If the AP is not where it should be, behavior, feelings, cognitive function, and health are affected. Below is from the work of Jon Whale and can be found at the Whale Medical website. Not taking the AP into account in diagnosis of medical and psychiatric dysfunctions because of the usual medical establishment control of the standard of care is just another example of how progress is held back in the name of greed. "Modern doctors" feel that recent advancements in pharmacology and surgery far exceed these old antiquated methods. It is my belief that they have been misled by these very profitable institutions and what really is happening is that medicine has gone off on a tangent, believing drugs and surgery are the future. Many of us in research believe that the future was already shown to us thousands of years ago. It could also be that laziness and that it takes a lot to time, which is money, to learn and practice something that may be better than what we were taught in school is holding us back.

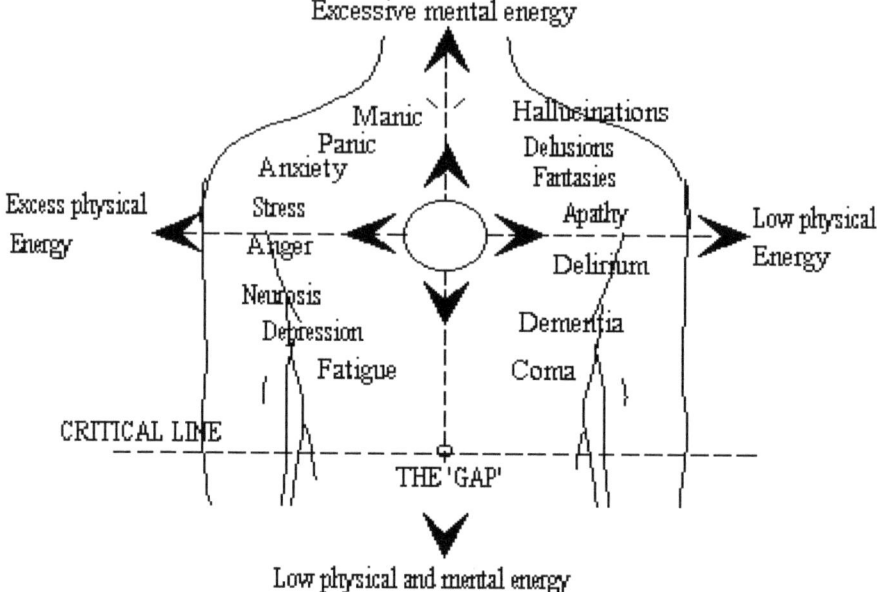

The following quotes the work of Dr. Jon Whale, a pioneer in this emerging field of medical diagnosis and treatment. If we can find a way to keep the establishment from stopping this new field, the cash cow of Big Pharma may lose a little weight.

THE SEVEN RULES OF THE HUMAN ASSEMBLAGE POINT

1. At the physical, emotional, atomic, and quantum levels, a human being is an independent oscillating energy field. All oscillating energy fields, by virtue of the fact that they are oscillating, must have an epicentre or vortex of the rotation. The epicentre of the human energy field is called the Assemblage Point.

2. The location and entry angle of the Assemblage Point with respect to the physical body dictates the shape and distribution of the human energy field.
3. The shape and distribution of the human energy field are directly proportional to the biological energy and activity of the organs and glands in the physical body, also to the quality of the emotional energy.
4. The biological activity of the organs and glands determines the position of the Assemblage Point, and thus the shape and distribution of biological energy throughout the physical body.
5. The location and entry angle of the Assemblage Point has a direct influence over the biological activity of all of the organs and glands including the brain and these have a direct influence on the location of the Assemblage Point.
6. The location and entry angle of the Assemblage Point regulates how we feel and behave. Disease also dictates the Assemblage Point location and entry angle.
7. The way we feel and the manner in which we behave, our state of health or disease, and our ability to recover are reflected in the location and entry angle of our Assemblage Point.

The idea that how we behave and how we feel might be beyond our rational control is largely unbelievable to most healthy people. Such people are extremely fortunate as they have a stable, near-central Assemblage Point.

This idea is acceptable and can be easily comprehended by anyone of us who has experienced any of the following:

1. Serious accident, bereavement, disease, fever, tragedy, chronic stress, or depression.

2. Distressed or oppressed childhood, rape or sexual assault, violent intimidation, kidnapping, abduction, enslavement.
3. Self laceration, mutilation or poisoning, attempted suicide, substance and drug indulgence, drug overdose, mental institution.
4. Mugging, robbery, burglary, fraud, identity theft.
5. Genocide, war, terrorism, homicide, torture, post military combat trauma, imprisonment.
6. Physical or psychological intimidation, interrogation, brainwashing.
7. Betrayal, financial or legal intimidation, blackmail, malicious divorce, bankruptcy, redundancy, home repossession, arrest, prosecution. Under any of these circumstances, many people can undergo a serious or seemingly permanent change of their mood or even a personality change. They may also develop physical symptoms and illness. This may eventually lead to more serious disease.

Any of these incident types can and do cause an involuntary shift of the Assemblage Point to a dangerous location.

Our Assemblage Point location fixes in a healthy, stationary, near-central position at around the age of seven if we are brought up in a stable home environment and positively identify with good mother- and father-figures.

But an unstable and displaced Assemblage Point is likely if we had a consistently negative relationship with our parents, a troubled background, or having a displaced upbringing. Genetic reasons or disease can similarly produce abnormal and unstable Assemblage Points.

Sufferers of an involuntary Assemblage Point shift downwards experience that 'something' deep inside them has changed. Although they can remember how they behaved and felt before the incident, returning to their former energetic and happy self is impossible for them. That indescribable 'something' deep inside all of us that can suddenly shift following an adversity, changing our whole perception of reality and our physical health, is the location and entry angle of our Assemblage Point.

If the Assemblage Point drops beyond a certain distance for example, with chronic fatigue, down to or below the liver area, despite what medications or therapies are employed, it is very difficult for the individual to recover his former health and state of being. This is because, without direct intervention, their Assemblage Point is most unlikely to return to its previous healthy location. Literally, the biological energy levels are too low, preventing recovery. Raising the Assemblage Point location and angle upwards, closer to the centre of the chest, is an essential consideration in such cases. Unfortunately, accepted orthodox medical diagnostic and management procedures do not take the patient's Assemblage Point location into consideration. In other words, a very successful method from the past takes a back seat to countless bogus and admittedly dangerous methods created by greed and bribery. Addiction has been proven to be correctable by reestablishing the location of the Assemblage point. What do doctors do? Their methods are extremely time-consuming and expensive with questionable results.

Gross misalignment of the Assemblage Point location is present in many diseases such as: depression, post natal depression, bipolar syndrome, paranoia, schizophrenia, drug and alcohol addiction, epilepsy, senile dementia, coma, Parkinsonism, toxicity, leukemia, cancer, auto immune deficiency syndrome, myalgic encephalomyelitis, multiple sclerosis, and many others. Many of these conditions are accompanied by compromised pathology of the patient's hematology and biochemistry.

Extreme locations to the right side of the chest with an acute angle are associated with extrovert psychotic behavior such as violence, bullying, rape, stalking, murder, terrorism or fanaticism. Dr. Jon Whale, in his book "Naked Spirit" describes a case of a pregnant lady addicted to drugs and alcohol whose assemblage point was found to be low and to the right. When it was relocated correctly the addiction desires no longer controlled her and both mother and child returned to health. How many victims of addiction could return to a normal life, saving the public enormous sums of money and eliminate the crime that goes with addiction? But the junk scientists would put it down as being not evidence-based. I would suggest that thousands of years of application eliminates the need to be evidence-based.

The field of Crystal Light Therapy has been used for thousands of years to reposition the AP and correct disease conditions, as well as emotional imbalances. Try to explain why this technology appeared in both eastern and western countries at the same time thousands of years ago. Now, modern technology is being applied with great success, its goal being able to make progress on the reestablishment of the original person that existed before the change. Traditionally, practitioners called shamans would apply a large crystal to the chest while giving a strong blow to the back. New technology has made it possible to eliminate the blow to the back using a gentle treatment called Theragem. On the web many more protocols are described as well as testimonials from respected professionals on the amazing results. If a new drug had come close to their results, the medical world would go crazy showing off.

Ultimately, shouldn't the ideal goal of medical treatment be to attempt to reestablish the original GOD created being? The being that existed before man screwed things up with processed or unnatural foods that cost less to produce, offering far less nutrition with a bonus of poisons called preservatives.

No worry for the selfish practitioners. There will always be plenty of irresponsible patients who refuse to pay attention to what really causes health problems. They will come to you.

A major deterrent to real progress is the arrogance of man thinking he is more intelligent than his predecessors. Not just in science, but throughout our left-brained dominant society, modern man thinks his thinking has improved to be better than our ancestors. Yes, we now have a tremendous number of conveniences, but are we more complete, fulfilled, and happy? I doubt we can construct any type of structure that will last over 2000 years. Our predecessors did.

The problem is that this "modern" crap is eliminating the human family unit, overpopulating a low-class society that cannot take care of itself and under breeding in the more intelligent classes. Preventing those from paying the price for not caring is counterproductive. Phony compassion for those who won't take part in helping themselves will ultimately help to create suffering for all. The above I learned in one of the first ecology classes given at UC Berkeley back when it was still an educational institution.

The world's present leadership, in its arrogance, thinks they know more than GOD. Due to the present day success of the greedy, politicians are dictating policies far beyond what their intelligence allows them to understand. Huge amounts are being spent on projects that they skim from, many times, doing far more harm than good. If they need a lot more money or power they can always start a war.

CHAPTER 5

LAZINESS: A MAJOR CAUSE OF MALPRACTICE

Getting an MD should be the BEGINING of one's studies!

When I was an undergraduate, some group of idiots came up with the idea that doctors should major in liberal arts fields so they "would be more well-rounded." One of many horrible results was the loss of the head of a baby's penis caused by a doctor using a Bovie to perform a circumcision. He didn't know the difference between a scalpel and electricity.

Not understanding the basic ways our body works due to lack of interest caused my late wife to require multiple(30) operations. Carol was struck by an out of control skier, breaking both legs, the right one in 17 places. The orthopedic, being unaware of the danger, opened the leg, realigned the pieces, and closed the wound. He did not replace the periosteum or help establish an ample blood supply and the wound reopened. Maintaining his lack of knowledge, he referred her to a plastic surgeon who was equally dumb. They also had little knowledge of pain control and I had to bring in a pain specialist, who, after days of pain, had it under control in an hour.

Why aren't all surgeons taught pain control?

Next I took my wife to UC Davis where the head doc said all of the previous operations, especially the first one, should never have been done. External fixation would have taken care of the fracture. There still was a problem getting the wound to close. I then took her to the best plastic surgeon I could find who concluded that all of the 10 plastic surgery attempts should not have been done because there was not sufficient blood supply. An artery was brought down from the abdomen and the wound finally closed. It was like 10 years of watching doctors play like children playing hospital. Carol lost what could have been the most fun years of her life, the 30's.

In my practice I make sure to know who the best in each field is and if that doc can do a better job, the patient comes first and receives a referral to one who can do it better.

As you may have guessed, more knowledge of the basic functions of the body would have prevented the above disaster. The rules regarding keeping one's medical license require many hours of continuing education per year at considerable time and expense. Big Pharm has the answer, stepping in and offering free or low-cost courses, sometimes in exotic places paid for. Having studied this way for some time, these doctors become symptom-treating, prescription-writing practitioners — no longer physicians.

I have found that there is much to be gained by me and my patients by reading literature of other scientific fields. By understanding these other areas of healthcare, I am better positioned to discover better methods of treatment of difficult conditions. Combining my methods with others, like acupuncture or hypnosis, can bring about relief that otherwise would not be accomplished. After a possibly unnecessary heart surgery, 10 days after my wife died, followed by therapy, my heart symptoms remained. I was referred to a hypnotist by an alternative practitioner and was free of these symptoms in two weeks. They were cortisol symptoms.

Once again, the lack of medical "outside the little box" education of the heart specialist had serious side effects. "Human Heart, Cosmic Heart" by Thomas Cowan, MD is a book I highly recommend to those who want to be proactive in their heart health.

Last year, I was referred a patient with pain in the parotid area of his left cheek. A neurologist was giving Botox shots in the cheek (treating the symptom). Upon my initial exam, just inspecting and palpating the entire area of the suspect cheek, I discovered a tumor that had extended into the left maxillary sinus. I ordered an MRI. The tumor was found to be entering the brain. It was huge, but luckily not metastatic. Extensive surgery was necessary, but we have a pain-free, tumor-free, living patient.

Physicians, when becoming specialists, to serve us best, must understand all other fields of medicine. New developments in the science of healthcare are coming so fast that a doctor can quickly find himself referring to far less effective treatment than he should have. Robotic surgery has replaced many surgeries with far faster recoveries and far more successful results, yet I still see surgeons who, not understanding robotics, do surgeries the old way.

My degree as a practitioner is in dentistry, but out of my craving of knowledge and my need for my own self-defense against dumb doctors, I have studied extensively most fields of medicine, probably saving my life or, at least, making my recovery much more complete. After Guillian Barre hit me last winter, doctors thought I was dying or at least would never walk or be normal again. Well, I was back 7 months later, better than before, working on patients and driving. I had to sneak in my own supplements and some real food and a little wine to make such a miraculous (the doctor's words) recovery.

I was dismissed on April 10, 2021. The only meds they sent me home with were blood thinners and statins. Finally, months later, I took it upon myself to study everything about GBS and how to repair the damage. About ten supplements are necessary to repair myelin and restore muscle damage created by this disease.

Once I began this repair regimen, improvement in everything (including numbness in my hands while sleeping which would wake me up) began to accelerate. If the goal of medicine were to get the patient well, instead of just pushing drugs, they would study what I studied or at least be aware of their shortcomings and refer me to one who specializes in the repair of what was damaged by the disease. Oh, but it is so much less trouble to leave my education to the pharmaceutical rep who drops my office and takes the free courses given by their companies. I think it is more than possible there have been new developments in basic sciences and other fields of medicine outside yours since you got your MD, but that would take some effort. No, what you guys did to me was give me some pills I might not need, and follow "the standard of care", not that you care.

In my opinion, the term "Standard of Care" should be abandoned. Now the Standard of Care for cancer is chemotherapy and radiation. An incredible man, Dr. Stanislaw Burzynski, developed a cure for a common very deadly brain cancer. Even though the existing "standard of care" had no cures, the FDA used this legal method to attempt to stop this cure.

Cured patients who had been given the death sentence by the "standard of care" appeared before congress and were able to get the FDA off their back. One glaring problem with his cure is the patient treats himself and the hospitals lose out along with Big Pharma. The Texas Medical groups took over and filed multiple suits which were stopped by the courts in just recent years. Senator John McCain might still be alive if he had been sent to Burzynski's clinic.

It is like the establishment is so lazy and greedy that they try to stop anything that would make them learn something or would eliminate the need for expensive drugs or procedures. Some of the research has been enhanced so much by quantum computers and it has become quite difficult to keep up with. I know the results are going to be so improved, that BIG PHARMA will be knocked off its throne hopefully forever. Doctors will then have to get off their butts and become true physicians and up-to-date surgeons. My own orthopedic surgeon had no knowledge of robotic surgery for carpal tunnel disease. Extensive recovery time was his way — took almost no recovery time robotically.

CHAPTER 6

THERE IS HOPE

Luckily, there still exists many good humans who have survived our educational system with an intact and active right brain and did not give in to the temptation of greed. I have the privilege of enjoying the friendship of several scientists and medical practitioners with these attributes.

Hopefully the swamp will be drained and the FDA, who presently is a major stumbling block to medical progress, will become honest and lobbies will no longer exist. All agencies need to be cleaned up. For no honest reason, Medicare will not pay for certain non-drug therapies like white laser and microcurrent therapy. The CDC is forcing dangerous, unproven, and worthless vaccines on us. Alternative cancer treatments with far fewer side effects are being used in Europe but not allowed in the USA. Stem cell treatment used in Europe is not allowed in the USA even if they are miraculous. Millions of innocent patients are suffering and dying due to the government, but there is a glimmer of hope being created by too many professionals standing up to the establishment. Too many for them to murder.

A leading cancer hospital is fighting to eliminate chemotherapy. It might be that because there are now so many doctors going into natural cures that do not need drugs, the strangle hold of Big Pharma has loosened. In my pain clinic, I have not used a drug in many years with far faster and more lasting results.

A few years ago, I went to Budapest to research out the use of a Russian device referred to as LifeStream Szoftver, Sensitiv Imago. Using discoveries mentioned in chapter II by Royal Rife, Albert Abrams and others use a computer based diagnostic tool which can identify the unique oscillation characteristics of the different organs of the body. It is showing great promise. If the organ being studied emits unusual or corrupted frequencies, little blue, red, or black triangles appear over that area on a screen in front of the patient. Ideal are green or yellow triangles. These areas can be treated to a minor extent with this device or medical treatment can be used. The patient merely places the left hand on a metal plate or holds a metal object, places earphones on, and watches a screen while every organ is viewed. What a great tool this would be in my practice to emphasize the need for cooperation and lifestyle changes. If you could see that your heart is in trouble clearly, chances are you would take the doctor's advice.

It is able to give an early warning especially for symptoms that are caused by an organ that is not in the area of that organ, such as colitis causing migraines or trigger point pain. A *good* physician is aware of this phenomenon and would like to rule out an organ in question before treating the symptom. This method would save countless expenses, time, and effort. Not good for the establishment.

I witnessed the results of this analysis in another patient. A friend of mine showed black triangles over the left anterior descending coronary artery. This early warning of a future heart attack could be treated with chelation therapy rather than bypass surgery. By the way, junk medicine does not believe in chelation, probably because there isn't big money in prevention. In this patient, I performed a further test that revealed she had a very low magnesium level. Supplementation reversed the problem. Most alternative physicians feel that anyone who has had bypass surgery should automatically be given a chelating agent, such as EDTA, after surgery. If given before, there might be no need for surgery. If Pfizer had not bought the Milano protein, and stopped its development, this problem would not have been there.

Another field that came from the past and is now performing miracles is Microcurrent Therapy. Again, the Russians came up with it, developing the Scenar, but some really bright guys in TEXAS refined it, creating an unbelievable and far more diversified device called the Avazzia. Instead of the three Scenar algorithms, the Avazzia has 53 algorithms, with a multitude of adjustments that can be made within each. One of the beauties of this device is that it includes eastern medicine such as acupuncture and Ayurvedic medicine, bringing back the ancient gifts of the past. I have been receiving training in the Avazzia methods for years and have been amazed, taking over cases prominent institutions have given up on and have been medicating or using a prosthesis to treat symptoms. When I was in Budapest,

I applied the Avazzia to patients with chronic tennis elbow, carpal tunnel, and knee pain. Consistently, when asked to move the limb, their mouth dropped open in amazement. Pain was gone for the first time in months or even years.

In a case of a chemotherapy in a breast cancer patient, I used vagus nerve stimulation to bring back her appetite and positive emotions. Even though the oncologist was impressed, when I suggested some other alternative medicine therapies that create patient comfort, he said it was not part of his protocol. I would like to suggest a very unpleasant protocol for such a closed-minded jackass.

One of the many other beauties of Microcurrent therapy is its use in acupuncture. When using acupuncture for anesthesia, the application of minute electric currents enhances the effects greatly. As Paul Dudley White recommended in the 1970s, that anesthesia, which kills thousands of Americans each year, should be replaced with acupuncture, where the patient can have conversation during surgery, get up and walk to bed. And we think we are advanced.

Another very encouraging new development that will hopefully be too fast for the present controllers of health care is the introduction of quantum mechanics. Much of it is far too advanced for these dummies to understand than undermine. Much faster and complete diagnosis of health problems are coming. Reintroduction of previously outlawed discoveries such as Rife's cure for cancer and TB may soon be possible. The addition of such advances is welcome as robotic surgery should quickly destroy the need for long hospital stays and recovery time.

I understand that the thought of replacing dishonesty, greed, and lust for power with integrity, sharing, and love seems an impossible dream. If man is to survive, we must make that dream a reality as soon as possible.

I am presently in the process of writing another book, this one on applying quantum mechanics to everyday life including one's health: *Born Again – a quantum leap into a life of fulfillment.*

CONCLUSION

First, in concluding, I would like a new specialty to be added to medicine — a superspecialist in understanding what our tissues need as food to accelerate healing. Being holistic in nature, I expect a lot of resistance. As you know, I suffered a very serious and debilitating syndrome called Guillian Barre in which the myelin sheaths on my nerves were severely injured causing my muscles to be paralized and my heart to possibly be damaged. I was released from the hospital with a blood thinner and a statin. When I was their "miracle" patient, they paid no attention to what I ate. It wasn't the hospital food. The doctors were not interested in the many supplements I was taking. There was no thought to what we should do to create the maximum repair of the damage done. What caused me to become what they called "a miracle"?

For several months, I stumbled and fell, requiring stitches, then I woke up and got on the internet to find what to add to my paleo diet that would help. Within days, after adding several supplements, my recovery accelerated and I, after two months, was no longer stumbling, falling, or having to hold on to things. I can now take long hikes and lift weights.

There are all kinds of dietary changes for brain damage and preventing brain damage. Dr. Colon Dong arrested over 10,000 cases of arthritis with diet only. MS has been reversed with supplements, diet, and exercise. And I even stopped a severe heart condition with Magnesium! I could go on almost forever on this subject, but look at all the money that docs and hospitals and the pharmaceutical industry would lose. They neeeeeed sick people!

Can you imagine how much the overall health of humanity would be improved if we had, not the current nutritionists, but a full PhD in cellular preservation and restoration? Today's nutritionists are still promoting whole grains and low-fat diets and vegetable oils. Some still promote milk, "the deadly poison."

To overcome the horrible "wrong turn" taken by most of the industries involved in health care, I suggest several of the following steps. First and most of all, do everything to create more awareness of the public to the health problems that the medical industry actually is responsible for. I am more than likely alive because of what I suggested in my book, *Why*:

1. Be proactive in your healthcare.
2. Do all you can to get our politicians back to representing the people.
3. Encourage our schools to require time each day in the classroom to teach health and physiology.

4. End all lobbying in the FDA and CDC. Demand that appointees in scientific areas are qualified.
5. Enforce anti-trust laws to prevent businesses from buying out newly-discovered or even old cures in order to control treatment of a disease.
6. Encourage the use of time-tested remedies. I cured a very large cancer in my dog with turmeric. Hydrogen peroxide and ozone are used in other counties quite successfully for decades with very few side effects.
7. When a food is found to exacerbate a disease, get it off the hospital menu.
8. Begin highly-funded research of everything about mitochondria. They are not only our sole source of energy. They produce apoptosis which destroys cells that are not functioning as the DNA demands through the RNA.
9. Install board of experts who review the "Standard of Care" so that the law is not so inclined to punish those who are trying harder, like Dr. Burzynski, curing brain cancer without hurting the brain.
10. Standardize a medical and dietary history for each specialty with pages to be submitted to a national data bank. With the new quantum computers' diagnoses and treatment and even possibly most important, the cause can be quickly identified.
11. Absolutely never allow politicians, unless they are practicing scientists, to make medical decisions.

A LAST THOUGHT

COULD SUBJECTIVE THINKING BE DESTROYING HUMANITY AND OUR ENVIRONMENT?

Many times, in his arrogance, man has the idea that he is smarter than GOD. One of the ways GOD prevented overpopulation and its horrible effects on this beautiful planet was the occurrence of epidemics. Those who are in the worst health and shape are usually the first to go and the survivors are generally those who are doing the most to be resistant. Our society, in its infinite wisdom, tries to interfere due to it being so kind and compassionate. **WOULD IT NOT BE MORE KIND TO LET SOME SUFFER A FEW DAYS OF ILLNESS FOLLOWED BY DEATH THAN HAVE EVERYONE SUFFER A SLOW DEATH FROM THE DISEASES OF OVER POPULATION?** Lack of food causing starvation and multiple long-term diseases caused by poor water and contamination, the loss of everything beautiful on earth and the emotional problems that would accompany this — I feel strongly this would be worse than death.

FOR ME, AND PROBABLY MOST, I WILL TAKE GOD'S WAY.

The End.

www.ingramcontent.com/pod-product-compliance
Ingram Content Group UK Ltd.
Pitfield, Milton Keynes, MK11 3LW, UK
UKHW022220230426